First Aid For Your Heart

A Guide To First Aid And Preventions

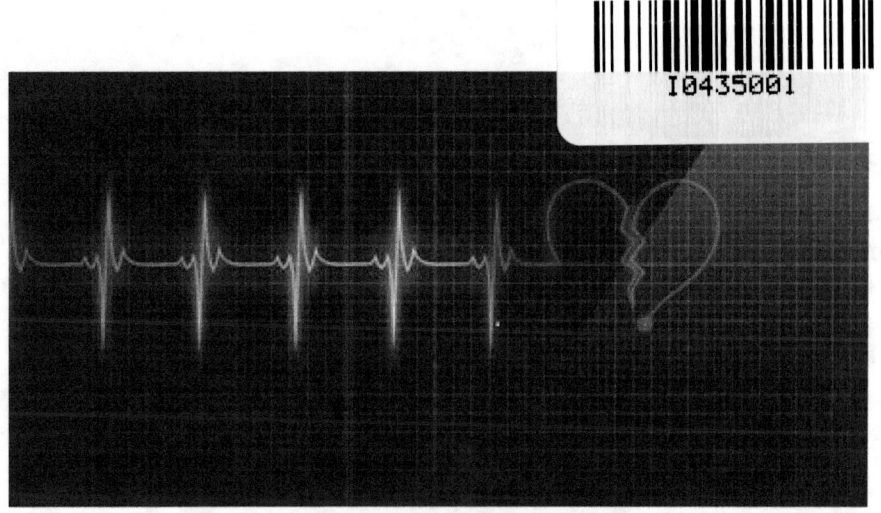

I0435001

Health Learning Series

M. Usman

Mendon Cottage Books

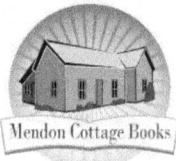

JD-Biz Publishing

Disclaimer

The information is this book is provided for informational purposes only. It is not intended to be used and medical advice or a substitute for proper medical treatment by a qualified health care provider. The information is believed to be accurate as presented based on research by the author.

The contents have not been evaluated by the U.S. Food and Drug Administration or any other Government or Health Organization and the contents in this book are not to be used to treat cure or prevent disease.

The author or publisher is not responsible for the use or safety of any diet, procedure or treatment mentioned in this book. The author or publisher is not responsible for errors or omissions that may exist.

Warning

The Book is for informational purposes only and before taking on any diet, treatment or medical procedure, it is recommended to consult with your primary health care provider.

Our books are available at
1. Amazon.com
2. Barnes and Noble
3. Itunes
4. Kobo
5. Smashwords
6. Google Play Books

Table of Contents

Preface

Your heart is the most important organ of your body. Its functionality gives us blood and oxygen, without which, no other organs can survive. Life knows no other means if your heart gives way. When we realize the vital importance of this organ we should also recognize our duties to keep it healthy and functioning perfectly. Yes, sometimes nature cannot be combated with, but self induced harshness on this asset of the body is our loss indeed.

Heart conditions, once deteriorated, require continuous precautions for the rest of the life with the fear of another attack dangling dangerously above your head. So we will tell you the better way, the precautions we can take up earlier in our lives to keep this tragic event at bay.

This book is about you recognizing what your heart is and provides you with knowledge of the symptoms of when its health is deteriorating in various forms. We provide you with health tips and, most essentially, the first aid steps if you witness a heart disease.

Once caught in a trap of heart disease, we add steps that you have to adopt, as now they will not be an option but will be an imposition upon you. So it is always better to keep things under your control rather than at the mercy of medicine or forced precautions.

Chapter 1 – Introduction

Your heart is undoubtedly the most crucial part of your body. It is the center of your cardiovascular system and is responsible for more or less everything that gives your body life. The transportation of oxygen and the success of your immune system all are dependent on the working condition of your heart. Keeping this heart up and running is highly relevant if you want a life of good health. Everything from the food you eat to the activities you partake affects your heart.

Heart disease is not a trivial matter and it is the leading cause of death among men and women in the United States of America. According to the center for disease control and prevention, a person in America suffers a heart attack every twenty five seconds. Another important thing to note is that most people perceive heart diseases to be a part of old age and are not worried about it in their younger age. This is an absolutely faulty approach to this risk, as it affects people in their twenties as well. More women die from heart attacks than breast cancer in their twenties, according to Dr. Noel Bairey Merz M.D of the women heart center Los Angeles. The heart attack rates in both men and women are rising sharply and we have to start taking actions at a very young age to prevent this disease from growing.

Chapter 2 - Understanding the problem

Let us start by understanding what exactly we mean by heart diseases and understanding its various types.

The heart is the center of the cardiovascular system. Through the body's blood vessels, the heart pumps blood to all of the body's cells. The blood carries oxygen, which the cells need. Cardiovascular disease is a group of problems that occur when the heart and blood vessels aren't working the way they should.

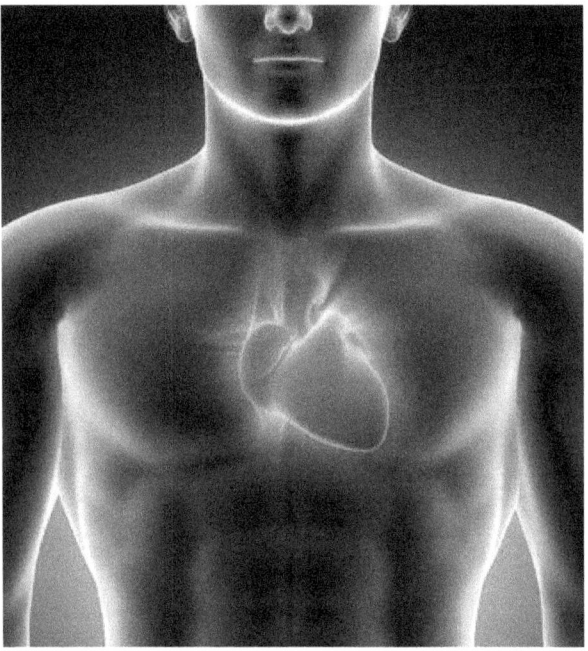

Here are some of the problems that go along with cardiovascular disease:

- Arteriosclerosis, also called the hardening of the arteries, arteriosclerosis means the arteries become thickened and are no longer as flexible.

- Atherosclerosis, is a build-up of cholesterol and fat that makes the arteries narrower so less blood can flow through. Those build-ups are called plaque.

- Angina, people with angina feel a pain in the chest that means the heart isn't getting enough blood.

- Heart attack, when a blood clot or other blockage cuts blood flow to a part of the heart.

- Stroke, when part of the brain doesn't get enough blood due to a clot or a burst blood vessel.

Symptoms of moderate to severe atherosclerosis depend on which arteries are affected. For example:

a. If you have atherosclerosis in your heart arteries, you may have symptoms, such as chest pain or pressure (angina).

b. If you have atherosclerosis in the arteries leading to your brain, you may have signs and symptoms such as sudden numbness in your arms or legs, difficulty in speaking, or drooping muscles in your face.

c. If you have atherosclerosis in the arteries in your arms and legs, you may have symptoms of peripheral artery disease, such as leg pain when walking.

d. If you have atherosclerosis in the arteries leading to your kidneys, you develop high blood pressure or kidney failure.

e. If you have atherosclerosis in the arteries leading to your genitals, you may have difficulties having sex. Sometimes, atherosclerosis can cause erectile dysfunction in men. In women, high blood pressure can reduce blood flow to the vagina, making sex less pleasurable.

If you think you have atherosclerosis, talk to your doctor. Also pay attention to early symptoms of inadequate blood flow, such as chest pain (angina), leg pain or numbness. Early diagnosis and treatment can stop atherosclerosis from worsening and prevent a heart attack, stroke or another medical emergency.

Causes of cardiovascular disease

While cardiovascular diseases can refer to different types of heart or blood vessel problems, the term is often used to mean damage caused to your heart or blood vessels by atherosclerosis, an accumulation of fatty plaques in your arteries. This is a disease that damages your arteries. Healthy arteries are flexible and strong. Too much pressure in your arteries can make the walls thick and stiff, and sometimes, restricts blood flow to your organs. This process is called hardening of the arteries (arteriosclerosis). Atherosclerosis is the most common form of this disorder. Atherosclerosis is often caused by an unhealthy diet, being overweight and smoking.

We shall now introduce you to various heart diseases and explain the symptoms and first aid treatments that you can safely adopt.

Chapter 3 - Heart arrhythmia

Heart arrhythmia is the scenario where the heart beats at an irregular pace or pattern. Sometimes more than a 200 beats per minute or sometimes as low as 50-60 beats per minute.

Causes of heart arrhythmia

Common causes of abnormal heart rhythms (arrhythmia) or conditions that can lead to arrhythmias include:

- Heart defects at birth

- Coronary artery disease

- High blood pressure

- Diabetes

- Smoking

- Excessive use of alcohol or caffeine

- Drug abuse

- Stress

- Some prescription medications and herbal remedies

In a healthy person it's unlikely for a fatal arrhythmia to develop without some outside influence, such as an electrical shock or the use of illegal drugs. The primary reason is that a healthy person's heart is free from any abnormal conditions that cause an arrhythmia, such as an area of scarred tissue.

However, in a heart that's deformed, the heart's electrical impulses may not properly initiate or travel through the heart, making arrhythmias more likely to develop.

Symptoms of Arrhythmias

The symptoms of arrhythmia are not too clear and sometimes your doctor may suspect arrhythmia before it even begins, through your routine medical checkups. However the symptoms arrhythmia does indicate are as follows.

- Feeling of skipped heart beats, fluttering in your chest.

- Pounding in your chest.

- Feeling dizzy or light-headed.

- Shortness of breath.

- Chest discomfort.

- Weakness

First aid for arrhythmia

Ventricular fibrillation is a type of arrhythmia that can be deadly. It occurs when the heart beats with rapid electrical impulses. This causes the ventricles to shake uselessly instead of pumping blood. Without an effective heartbeat, blood pressure plummets, cutting off blood supply to your vital organs. A person with ventricular fibrillation will collapse within seconds and soon won't be breathing or have a pulse. If this occurs, follow these steps:

- Call 911 or the emergency number in your area.

- If there's no one trained in cardiopulmonary resuscitation (CPR), provide hands-only CPR. Make sure that the chest compressions, of about 100 a minute, are continued until paramedics arrive. To do chest compressions, push hard and fast in the center of the chest. You don't need to do rescue breathing.

- Find out if an automated external defibrillator (AED) is available nearby. These portable defibrillators can deliver an electric shock that will resume heartbeats. These are available in a wide range of places, such as in airports and shopping malls. You can also purchase one for your home and no particular training is required for it. They're programmed to allow a shock only when appropriate and not otherwise.

Chapter 4 - Angina

Angina is the pain that comes from the chest region. Every year, around 20,000 people suffer from this problem in the United Kingdom. Unlike the common believe that angina hits more men and old people, this condition is rather common in women and younger people.

If you have angina, one or more of the coronary arteries are narrowed. Now what happens is that the amount of blood supply is reduced to a part of your heart muscle. The blood supply is ample when you are resting, but while exercising or running too fast, the heart rate increases and as a result you need more oxygen. The extra blood that your heart requires cannot pass through the narrowed arteries and there occurs a pain in the chest region. In simple words, the energy demands on the heart outpace the blood supply. There are different forms of angina and in more severe forms of angina the arteries are clogged to such an extent that chest pain appears when you're resting and doing no physical exertion.

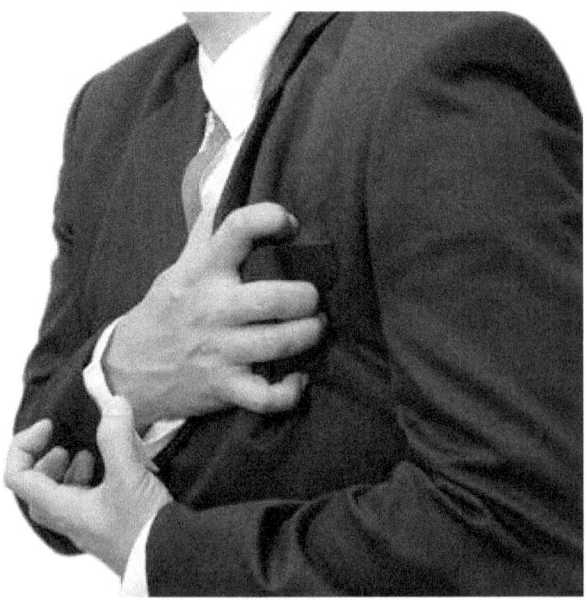

Symptoms

The most common symptom of angina is pain, ache and an uncomfortable feeling on the front of the chest when you overexert yourself. Climbing stairs or walking against strong wind is example of overexertion. A painful sensation may also be felt upon the arms, jaw, neck and stomach. Some people neglect pain in the central, upper part of the stomach and they confuse it with indigestion. But, it can be a lethal mistake that you can make. This pain can be actually be due to angina. Pain felt during angina is not long lasting and usually within the ten minutes of resting you may feel that the pain is receding.

First aid

The first step to take while facing any heart problem is to stop whatever activity had initiated the pain and rest immediately. Remaining calm is a vital part as well, because it will make your heart beats more stable. Call 911 or the valid emergency number of your area.

Step 2 is to lie down in a comfortable position and keep your head up. Try to normalize your breathing. It will help you recover, as well as diverting your attention from the pain.

Step 3 is to chew an adult aspirin (make sure that you are not allergic to aspirin before taking this step). Please make sure that you do not chew more than 1, as prolonged or increased usage will do more harm than good.

Step 4 is when you have had angina before ONLY in this case use sublingual nitro-glycerine and visit the emergency room.

Chapter 5 - Bradycardia

Bradycardia means that your heart is beating very slowly. Generally, a heart rate of 60 to 100 beats a minute while at rest is considered normal. If your heart beats less than 60 times a minute, it is slower than normal.

For some people, a slow heart rate does not cause any problems. It can be a sign of being very fit. Healthy young adults and athletes often have heart rates of less than 60 beats a minute.

In other people, bradycardia is a sign of a problem with the heart's electrical system. It means that the electrical pathways of the heart are disrupted. In severe forms of bradycardia, the heart beats so slowly that it doesn't pump enough blood to meet the body's requirements. As a person ages, the electrical system of the heart often doesn't function normally.

Bradycardia may be caused by the process of aging or if a person has taken up a disease that damages the heart's electrical system.

Symptoms

A very slow heart rate may cause you to:

- Feel dizzy or lightheaded

- Feel short of breath

- Feel tired

- Have chest pain

- Have trouble concentrating

- Have a pulse weaker in intensity and fewer in number.

Conventional treatment

If you have no symptoms, medical treatment may not be necessary. Bradycardia can be caused by medication, which if it can be stopped, may cause your slow heart rate to normalize. However, because bradycardia is usually related to problems with cardiac conduction, the only method currently available to increase heart rate is with the use of a pacemaker.

Temporary pacemakers can be used. Permanent pacemakers become necessary when bradycardia is an irreversible condition. Pacemakers can also be used to treat fainting spells, congestive heart failure, hypertrophic cardiomyopathy, and other conditions where a consistent heart rate is imperative. A pacemaker implantation is a simple outpatient procedure.

Chapter 6 - Heart attack

Heart defects or diseases usually develop while the baby is still in the womb. As the heart begins to develop the defects may begin to form. Medical conditions and some genes may be responsible for this. It may also develop in adults. As you age, the structure of the heart also changes and defects may be formed at this stage.

Infections like pericarditis, myocarditis and endocarditis are caused by four common irritants

- Bacteria cause endocarditis by entering through our bloodstreams. It enters the bloodstreams through everyday activities like eating or brushing our teeth. Our oral heath encourages the flow of such bacteria. Intravenous drug abusers are also more prone to get this condition.

- Viruses can cause myocarditis and other problems. They are usually associated with sexually transmitted infections.

- Parasites like trypanosoma cruzi are transmitted by insects and they can form a disease known as Chaga's disease.

- Some medications, like antibiotics such as penicillin, may create toxic or allergic reactions. Cocaine also may contribute to it. The needles used to transmit these medication can transmit these viruses that may cause heart infections.

Symptoms of a Heart Attack

- Pressure, discomfort, pain in chest, arm ,or below the breastbone.

- Discomfort flowing to the back, arm, throat, or jaw.

- Indigestion and choking feeling.

- Sweating profusely, nausea and dizziness.

- Weakness, anxiety, and shortness of breath.

- Irregular or rapid heartbeat.

During a heart attack, symptoms last thirty minutes or longer and are not relieved by rest or oral medications. Symptoms may start as a mild discomfort which progresses to immense pain.

What do you do in the scenario of a heart attack?

The following are details to be followed when having a heart attack or witnessing one.

The immediate step is to call 911 or your local emergency helpline number. Heart attacks are an issue that requires immediate medical attention and there are steps to be taken that only a medical expert can deal with. If you don't have access to medical services, have someone drive you over to the hospital immediately. Only as a last resort, you are allowed to drive yourself, otherwise this is an unnecessary risk that you have to avoid at all costs.

Unless you have been forbidden to take aspirin, immediately chew or swallow one. If this is another episode of heart attack and you have been prescribed nitro-glycerine then use that. DO NOT TAKE SOMEONE ELSE'S NITROGLYCERIN. Begin CPR if the person becomes unconscious. If you are not aware of the proper methodology, doctors recommend mouth to mouth rescue and performing only chest compressions.

Chapter 7 - How to perform a CPR (cardiopulmonary resuscitation)

There are two aims of CPR; firstly, it artificially pumps blood out of the heart and around the body. The chest compressions provide this action. Secondly, artificial flow of oxygen to lungs is initiated; artificial respiration performs this task. Now we shall explain how these separate actions work.

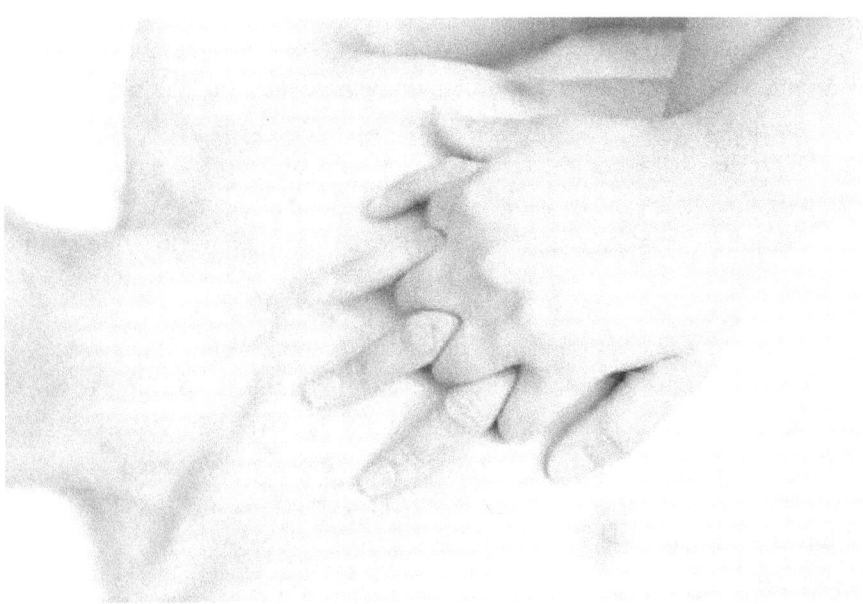

Chest compressions

❖ Kneel by the side of the victim (on the right side of the victim).

❖ Place the heel of one hand in the centre of the chest of the victim (the breastbone).

❖ Place the heel of the other hand on top of the first one and join your fingers together.

❖ Keeping your elbows perfectly straight bring your entire bodyweight down to ensure a vertical press.

❖ Be firm in pressing down and make sure the downwards movement is of around four to five centimeters. Make sure that your elbows remain locked and the force comes from your back and entire arms. Relax and then repeat the compression. After each compression, release pressure but make sure that the contact of the hands and the breastbone is not relaxed.

❖ Try to achieve a target of 100 compressions per minute. Be loud in your count.

❖ Do this around thirty times then move on to artificial respiration twice and continue with this ratio.

Artificial respiration

❖ By tilting the head of the victim back, raise his chin.

❖ Pinch the nostrils shut with two fingers to prevent leakage of air.

❖ Take a deep breath and close your own mouth over the other person's mouth. Cover the victim's mouth first with a piece of cloth.

❖ Make sure you breathe slowly into the other person's mouth; it takes approximately two seconds to properly inflate the chest. If the chest raises properly it means that you're doing it properly.

❖ Repeat this process again.

❖ Make sure you check if the victim's chest rises when you breathe into him, if it does, all is well, but if it doesn't, try to hold the head back further and lift the chin higher.

Simultaneous performance of CPR and artificial respiration

Although it is difficult if previously not practiced, try to get some help and do both these activities simultaneously. The ratio should be kept at 30 compressions to 2 artificial respirations. If breathing initiates but the person does not regain consciousness, then roll them gently over to their side in the position of recovery. This way mucus or vomiting can get out easily and will not obstruct their breathing.

Chapter 8 - Post heart attack, precautions for life

Exercise is now your best friend. It will improve your cardiovascular health. Keep in mind that the intensity of this exercise will vary for the different level of heart attack you had, so always select the program with consultation of your doctor. A trained clinician will work with you and your healthcare provider will develop a program that is safe for you. The fitness and physical limitations will all be incorporated in that program. Walking, jogging, cycling, rowing, and climbing are some examples. Always remember that the warm up and the cool down phases of exercises are the most important. In any exercise that you undertake, especially if it involves heart problems, you have to be extra careful about these two stages.

Factors you need to start reducing immediately

Say no to smoking and say it now. The risk of getting another heart attack decreases by half if you quit smoking. Going to group therapy sessions, using nicotine patches, gum, or nasal spray can be helpful in attempting this quit.

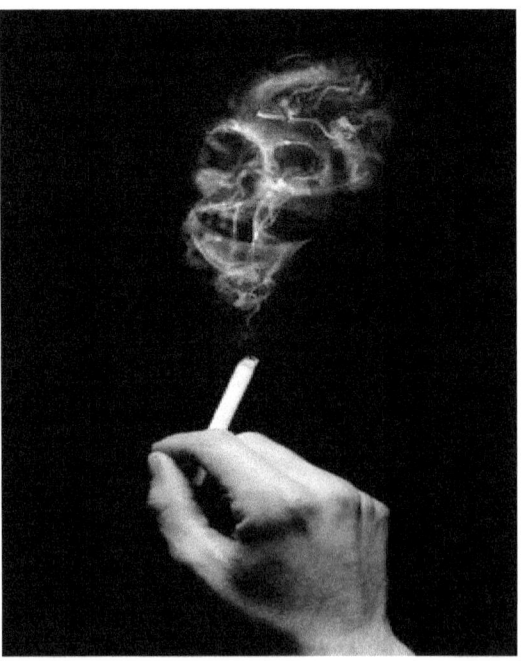

High blood pressure is a nuisance for a heart patient, so use the prescribed medication regularly and take a leaf out of our book and use some of our helpful tips and try to incorporate them in your daily life.

Proper medications should be taken at the advice of your doctor to keep your cholesterol levels low after the heart attack.

If you suffer from diabetes, then you are at a higher risk of developing complications after a heart attack. Tight blood sugar control is what's necessary for you now, and it can be achieved by losing weight, exercising, and taking insulin or other oral medication.

A registered dietitian is what you need. He is the best person to consult about precautionary diets that you should take to reduce cholesterol and blood sugar. He will be able to recommend diets, meal portions, and ways to reduce bad diet.

It is not uncommon to hear people going into depressions after a heart attack. You fear that you have to limit yourself now and of course too many restrictions and precautions do not make you feel so good. Therefore, individual or group therapy can be helpful for you so that your health problems do not flow into your family or your marriage.

Chapter 9 - Starting off healthy

Making a healthy start to life can make you relieved of problems that may arise in the future. Better choices and habits developed at younger ages are a blessing for tomorrow. Therefore, we are emphasizing to our children of today about getting into healthier habits and you have to contribute by following these duties to ensure a healthier future for them.

- Being a good role model is the best way to start off. No one is perfect and everyone has some weaknesses, but it is absolutely essential that we keep our weak side hidden from the younger generation and appear a model of perfection in their sight. If the kids see you eating right and being physically active that's perfect. Sending a good message is really important.

- Be positive in front of your kids, it is best for them to see the bright and optimistic side of the future and be full of high spirits.

- Plan group activities for your families and do not only include board games, though they should certainly be there too. Examples of such activity maybe riding bicycles, going to the beach for a swim, or anything that includes physical activitiy.

- Set small targets to achieve personal fitness. These targets will help your motivational level when you notice that you are achieving something. Setting unrealistic targets generally depresses a person.

- Television, video games, and computer times should be limited. Excessive use of that will mean less physical activity and more time on the couch with snacks.

- Encourage sports your child chooses or shows his/her interest in and help him in getting trained so that he can learn better and pursue it and remain fit.

- Make dinner time a family meal. This will insure proper diets and the likes and dislikes of your kids will get noticed by you and you can plan on how to incorporate healthier food in their systems.

- Keep monitoring your family and stay involved in their eating habits and physical activities, as this is the age where kids don't know what's best for them, and checks by parents are important for their health.

Chapter 10 - Keeping a healthy heart

We all know now how important our heart is, and to keep it working and fit is therefore an absolute necessity. Gladly there are a few basic ways we can cut down the chances of getting a heart disease. Having a good diet, drinking moderate alcohol, exercising daily to keep a normal body weight, and saying no to smoking can reduce your chances of getting a heart problem by 92% according to a Swedish study.

However, you might say okay these are very broad things and not all of them can be achieved or maintained overnight. You are correct if you think that, and we are going to provide you with numerous healthy tips. Try each of them one after the other, giving a day to each and carry on following as many tips as you like.

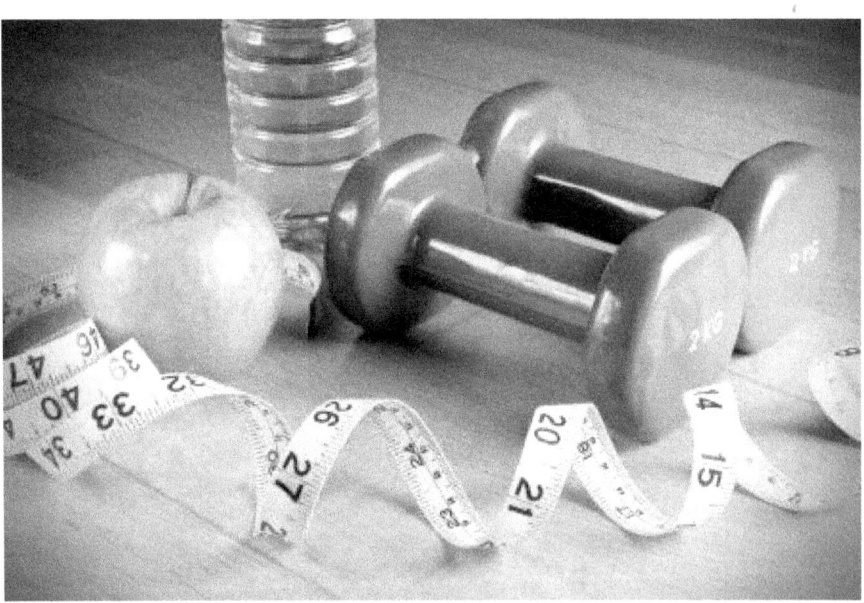

✓ Drink green tea. Green tea has several antioxidants that lower your cholesterol levels and can even reduce your blood pressure.

✓ Read food labels. When it comes to your heart health don't let the fats you consume exceed 30% of your calories intake. More importantly, make most of your fat from the healthy sources like olive oil, nuts, avocado, salmon, and walnuts. Avoid Tran's fat, as these fats are found in the cookies and other baked goods. We know they are hard to resist, but try to restrict them to 1% of your daily intake.

- ✓ Use olive oil in your food preparation. It reduces the risk of cancer and other chronic diseases like Alzheimer's. Substitute it for butter and margarine and drizzle it on salads and even in baking.

- ✓ Get an extra hour of sleep. When a person is sleep deprived his body releases stress hormones that constricts the arteries and creates inflammation. If you particularly feel tired or require an afternoon nap then you are most likely to be sleep deprived.

- ✓ Fiber up your diet. Load your meals with whole grain breads and toss beans into your salads. Aim for 25-30 grams of fiber daily.

- ✓ Make fish your favorite meat. Salmon and anchovies have omega-3 fatty acids that help your heart in maintaining a steady rhythm. One serving a weak will greatly help your heart health.

- ✓ Start your day with a glass of juice. Orange juice has folic acid that helps in lowering the levels of homocysteine, which is linked with a higher heart attack risk. Grape juice has potent antioxidants that discourage red blood cells from clogging together and blocking up the artery.

- ✓ Increase your veggies. Make vegetables at least 50% of your meal portion. Try to add broccoli, Brussel sprouts, and cabbage as they are known to be heart savers.

- ✓ Make nuts your favourite snacks. Don't overdo that though, otherwise you'll find yourself with a few extra pounds.

- ✓ Make a 20 minutes' walk part of your daily routine.

- ✓ Alter your bread spread. Olive oil is ideal for that, but if you want to pick another make sure it's the ones that have a cholesterol lowering sterol.

- ✓ Add flaxseed in your life. Sprinkle it over your daily yogurt, cereal, or salad as it also reduces the blockade in your arteries.

- ✓ Do daily ten to fifteen minutes of stretching as it will help in keeping your muscles flexible and your arteries pliable.

- ✓ Use soy to lower your cholesterol levels. It's best to avoid processed foods like chips and patties and soy supplements.

- ✓ A clove of garlic a day reduces the risk of heart attack in three ways. Firstly, it prevents blockage in arteries, secondly it reduces arterial damage and lastly it prevents cholesterol from lining the arteries that makes them narrow and blockage becomes more likely.

- ✓ Find fun ways to burn calories. Apart from your regular workout find more ways to burn calories; these may include dancing around while doing your chores or shooting hoops with your kids.

- ✓ Assess your stress levels. Spend time with people around you. Participate in group activities or sports that make you happy.

- ✓ Meditate for 5-10 minutes on daily basis. Simply close your eyes and take yourself away from every worry and see the storm of stress off.

- ✓ Keep in touch with faith. Even if you are not regular, do something for charity, as it will help cleanse your soul and you will feel at peace.

- ✓ Keep your loved ones close. Having strong ties with your family and your loved ones reduces anxiety and pressure. Promote family gatherings and have a sit-down dinner at least once a week.

- ✓ Fish oil and vitamin D are your saviours from heart diseases. Fish oil has omega 3 fatty acids that help in stabilizing the electrical system of your heart and reduce blood pressure. Vitamin D deficiencies can create heart risks and increases the chances of the development of diabetes.

- ✓ Keep a happy marriage. Married couples have a buffer against heart diseases (if you are happily married that is) couples who fight tend to have a higher blood pressure than average. Find little ways to keep away from the fights and that will help you find stress free happy life.

✓ Have a nip of a little dark chocolate daily. It will help in keeping the blood pressure in check. But do not take too much of the chocolate.

✓ Avoid passive smoking. If you don't smoke that's good, but also avoid staying too close to the ones who smoke next to you. This has harmful effects on your body as well.

✓ Eat loads of bananas. This has potassium which is excellent for your blood pressure.

✓ Cut down on your sugar intake. Large amounts elevate your blood pressure and reduce the production of nitric oxide, a gas that helps in relaxing and dilating the blood vessels.

✓ Laugh more. Seriously this will help in everything and every aspect of life will seem better.

Conclusion

Heart diseases are not contagious. There are some factors that you can control and some which you can't. Getting older, some people in your family having heart issues, maybe your parents, can have a genetic part to play and these are the factors beyond ones hands. However, other activities that we have discussed in detail like smoking, being overweight, and a lack of exercise are all issues that are within our reach and thus can be controlled.

References

http://www.mayoclinic.org/diseases-conditions/heart-arrhythmia/basics/symptoms/con-20027707

http://basicfirstaid.ca/importance-understanding-arrhythmias/

http://www.emedicinehealth.com/hardening_of_the_arteries/page7_em.htm#self-care_at_home

http://medpapers.wordpress.com/2013/01/07/knowledge-of-coronary-heart-disease-first-aid-memo-2/

http://www.webmd.com/first-aid/angina-pectoris-treatment

http://www.patient.co.uk/health/angina-leaflet\

http://www.emedicinehealth.com/bradycardia_slow_heart_rate-health/article_em.htm

http://www.liveto110.com/abnormal-heart-rhythm-bradycardia/

Author Bio

Muhammad Usman is a distinguished medical graduate of Allama Iqbal medical college (AIMC). He is a professional writer who has been in the field for more than 4 years. During this time he has produced 10,000+ articles, blogs and eBooks on various niches related to diseases, health, fitness, nutrition and well-being. He is a regular contributor to several journals related to medicine and surgery. He is the editor of several journals and newspapers.

Check out some of the other JD-Biz Publishing books

Gardening Series on Amazon

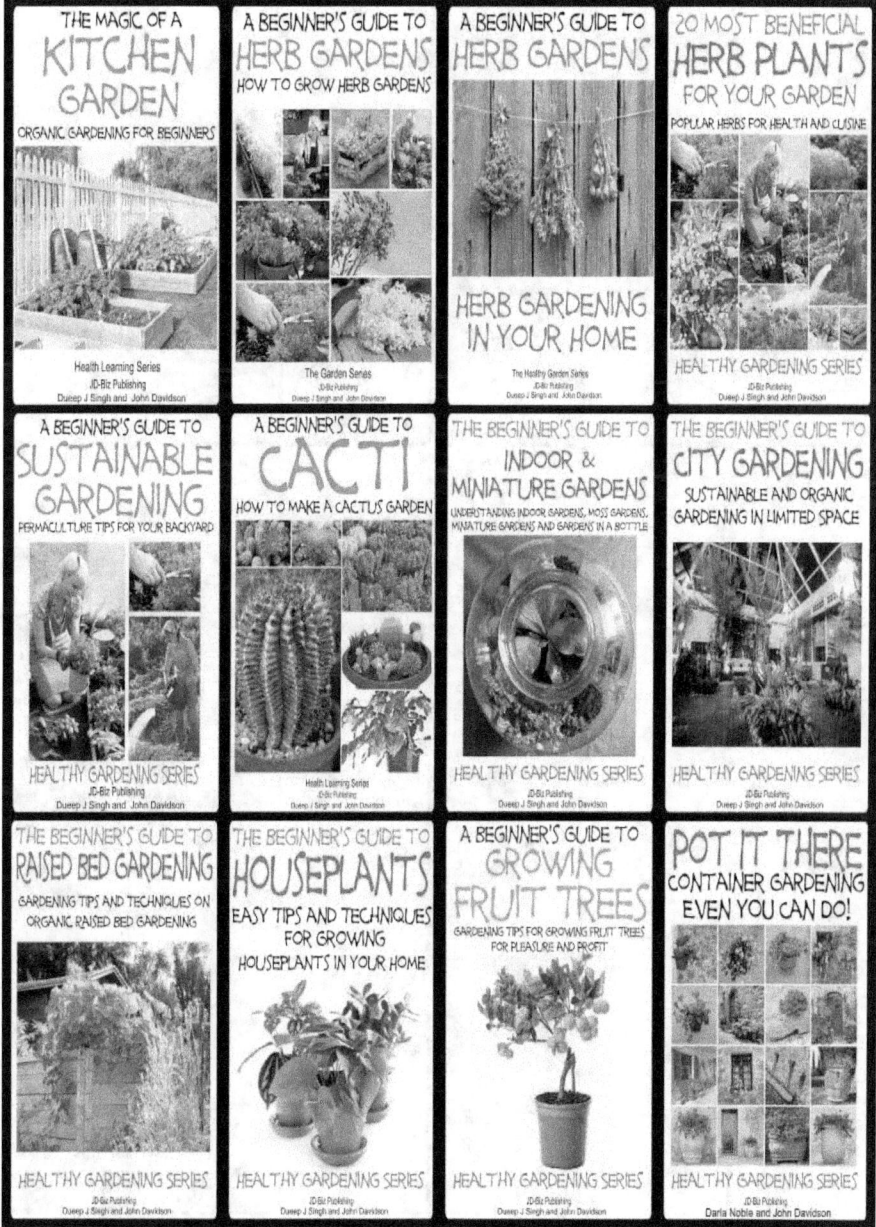

Health Learning Series

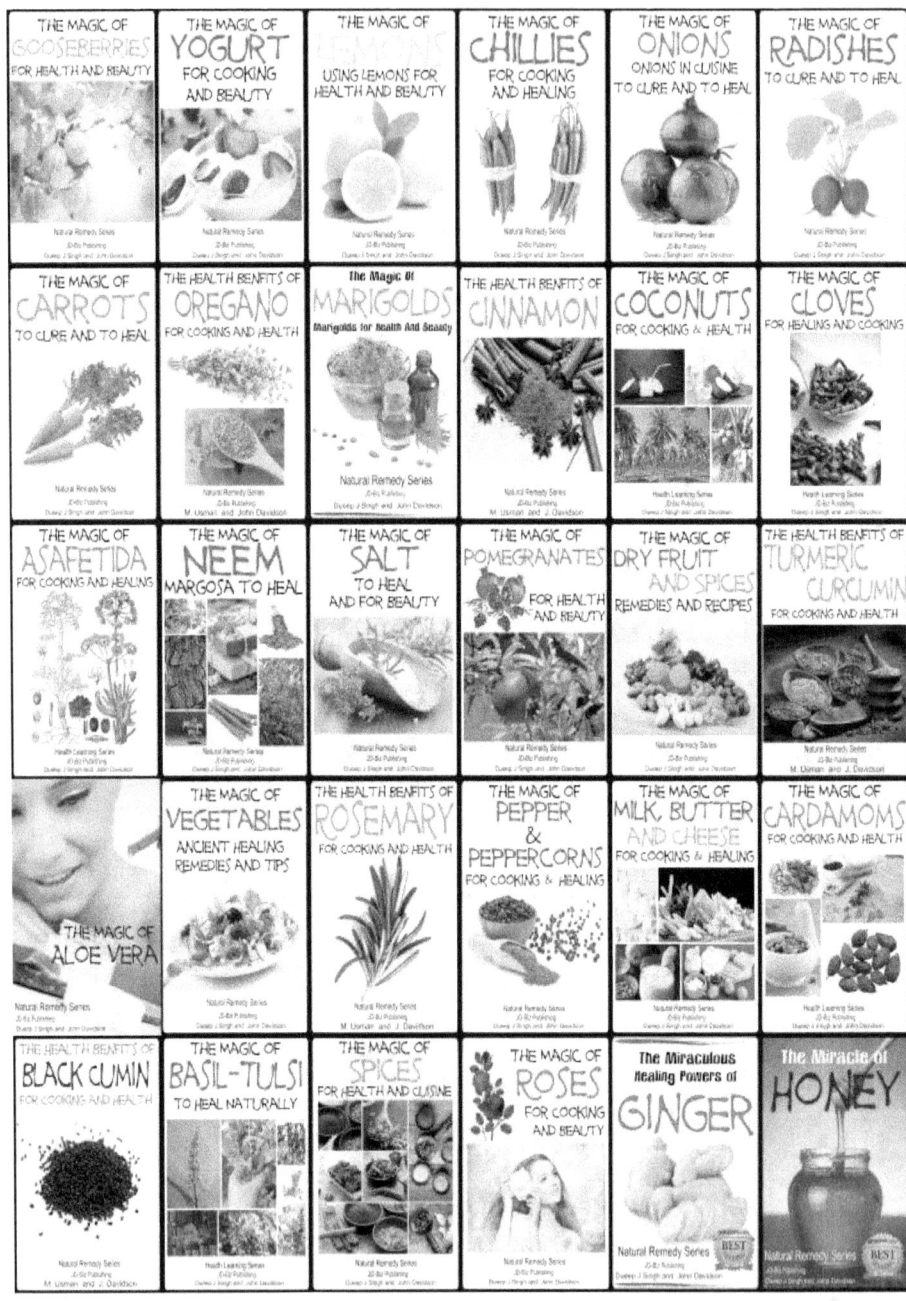

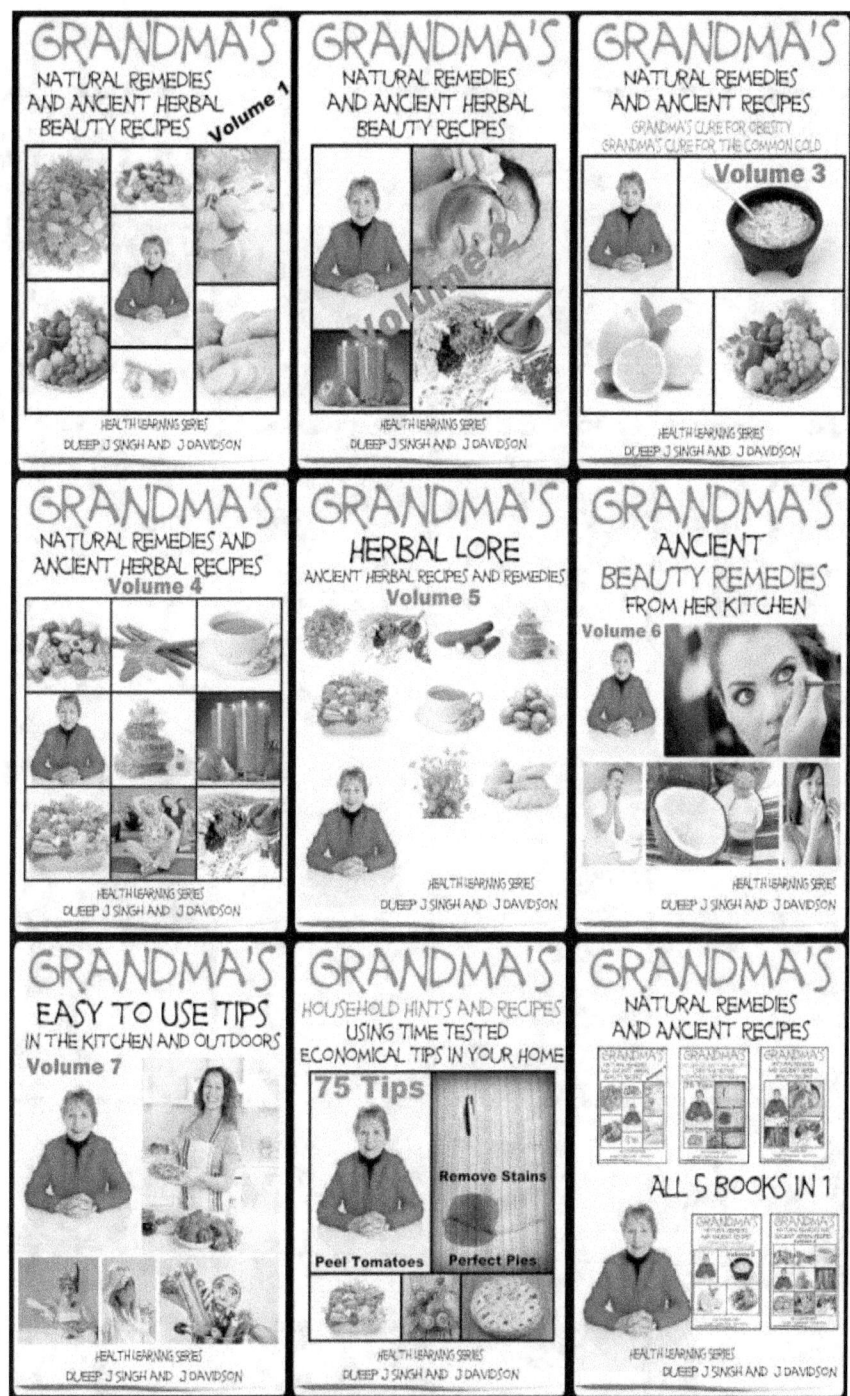

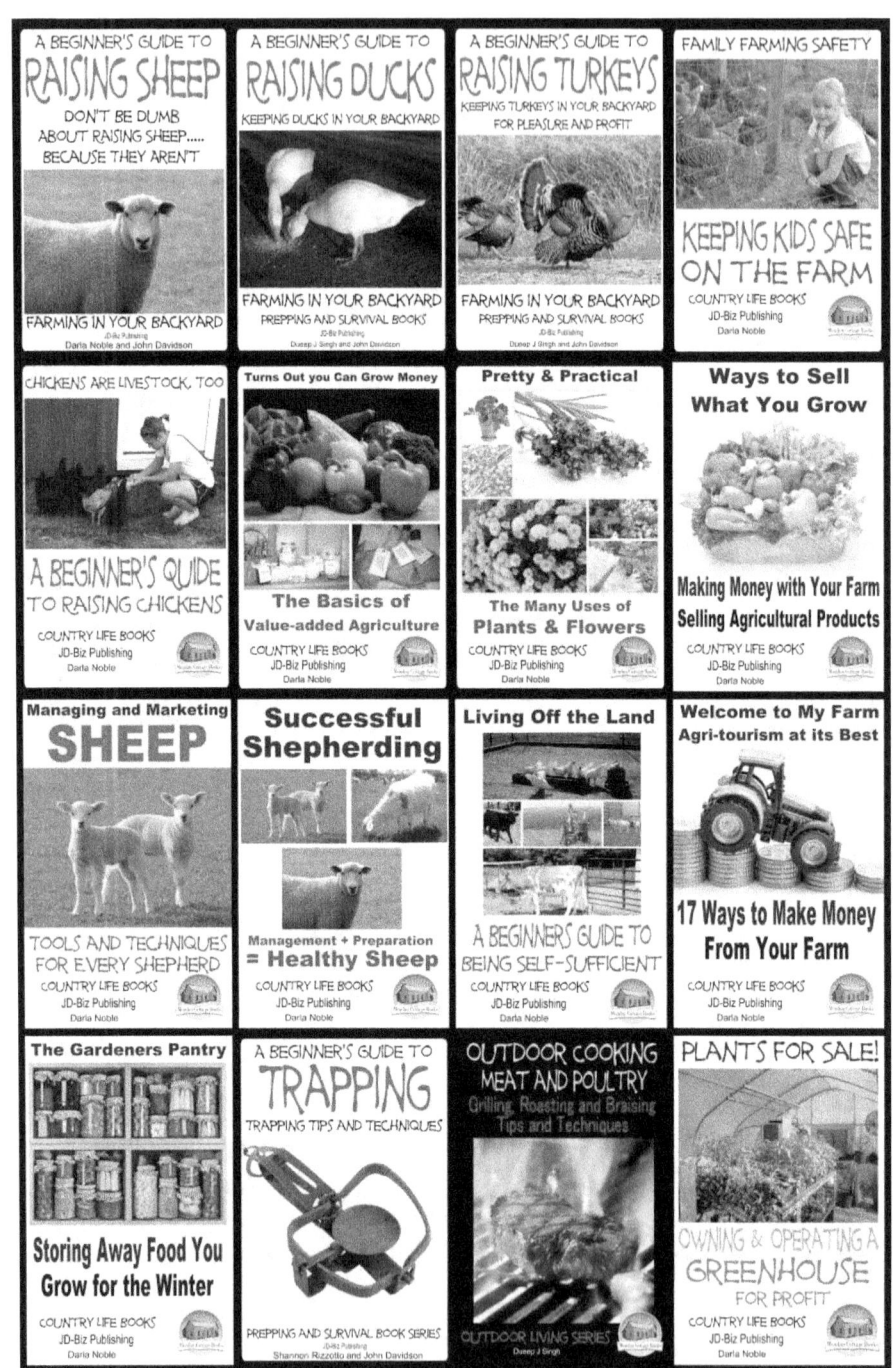

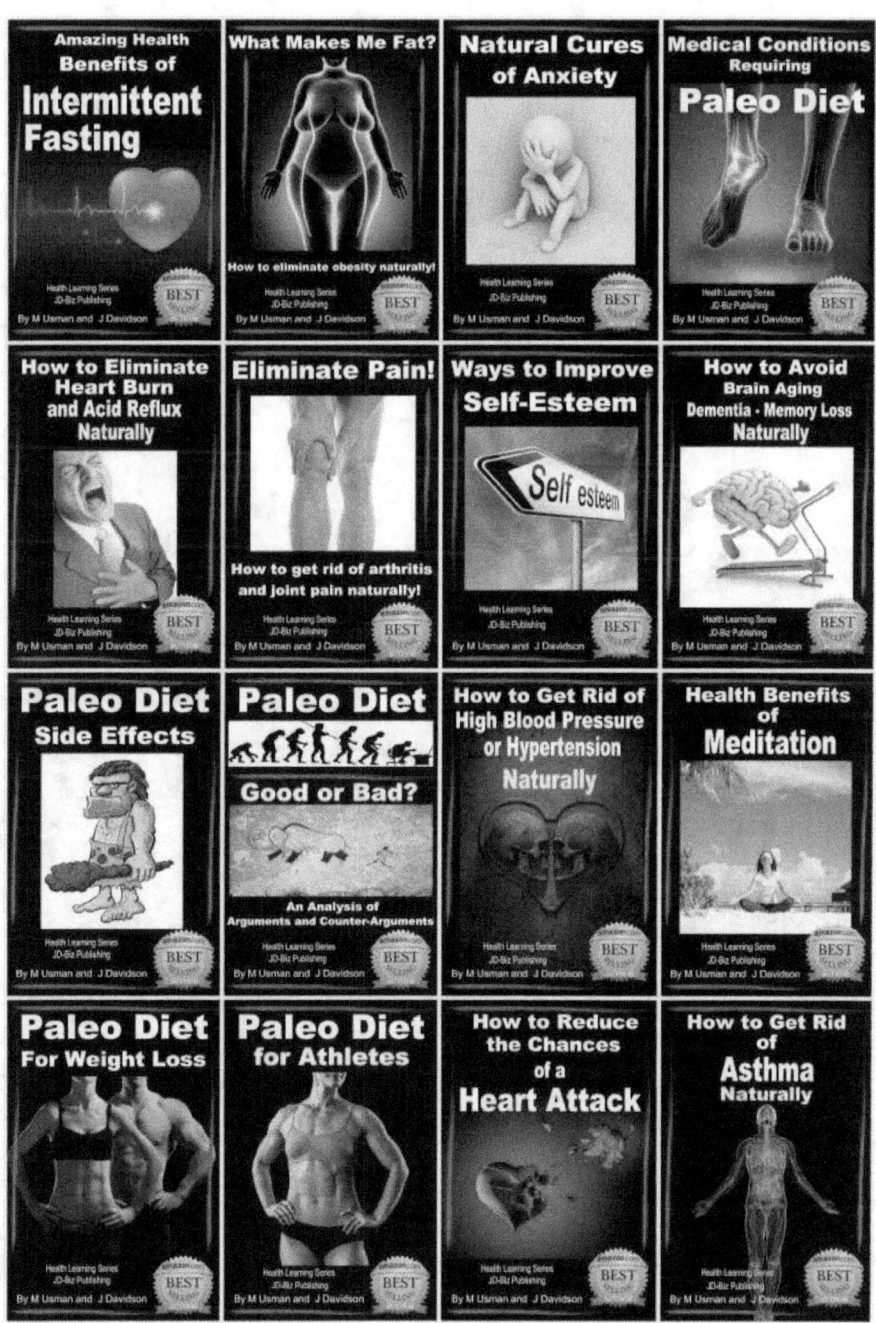

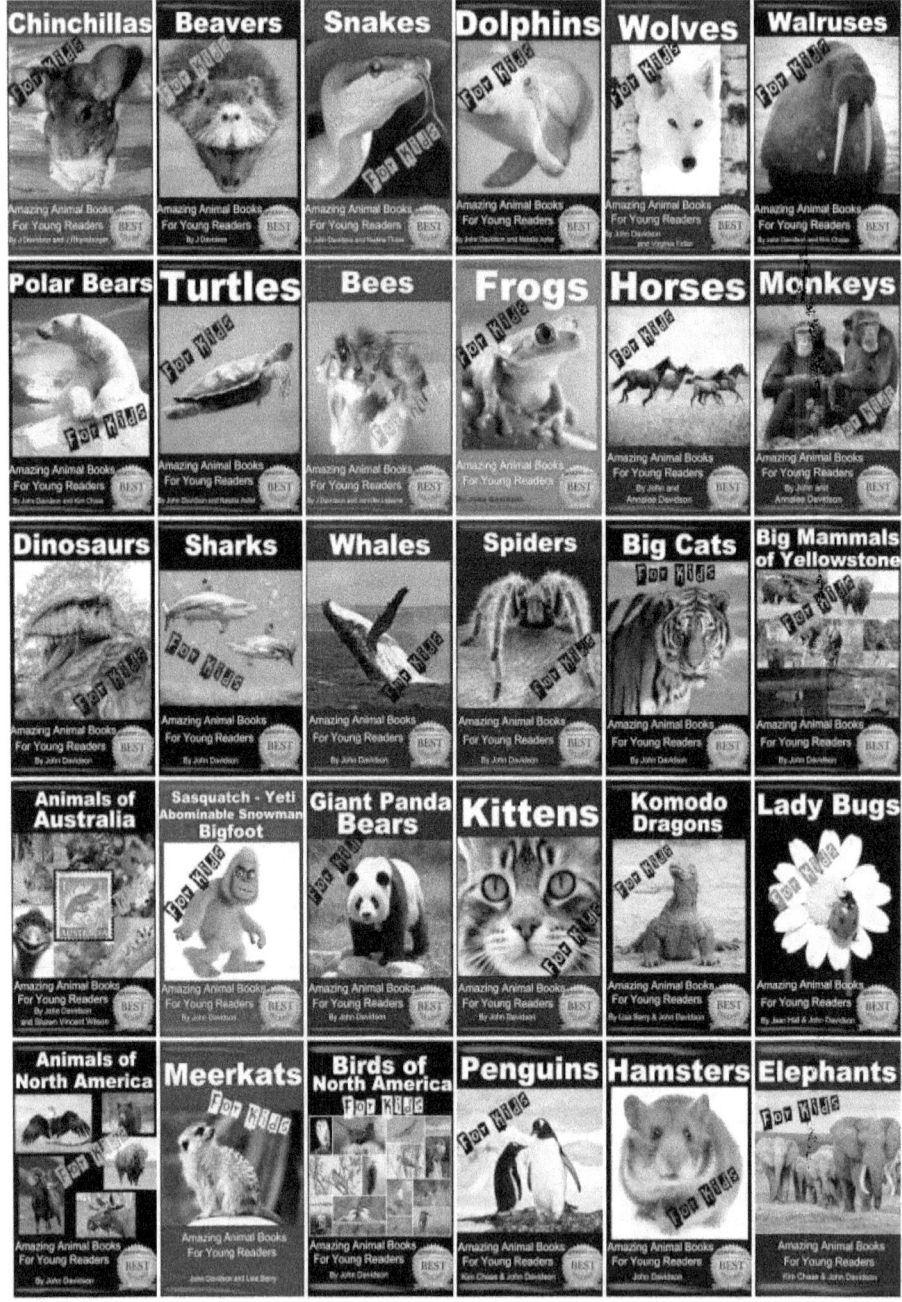

Learn To Draw Series

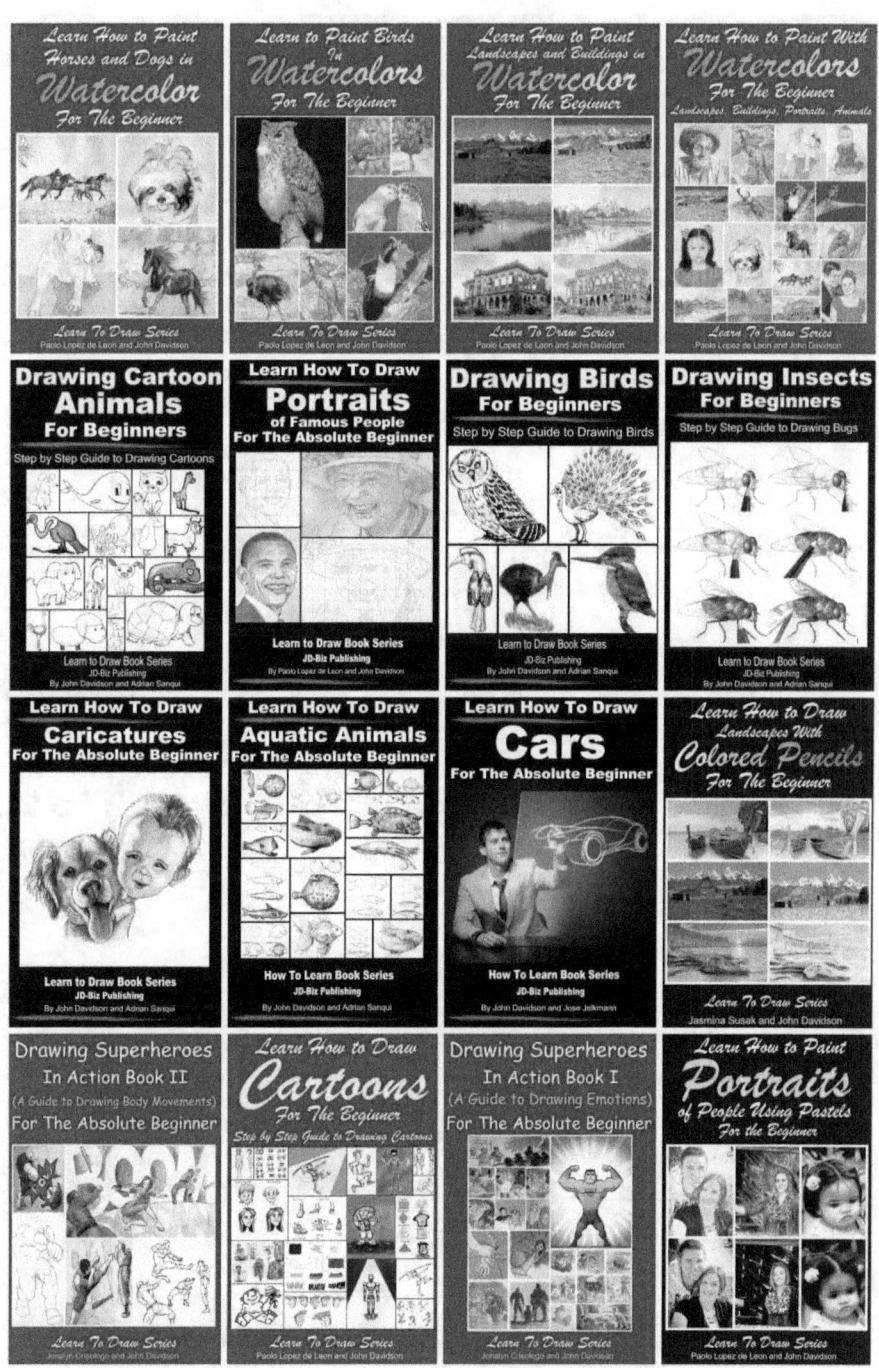

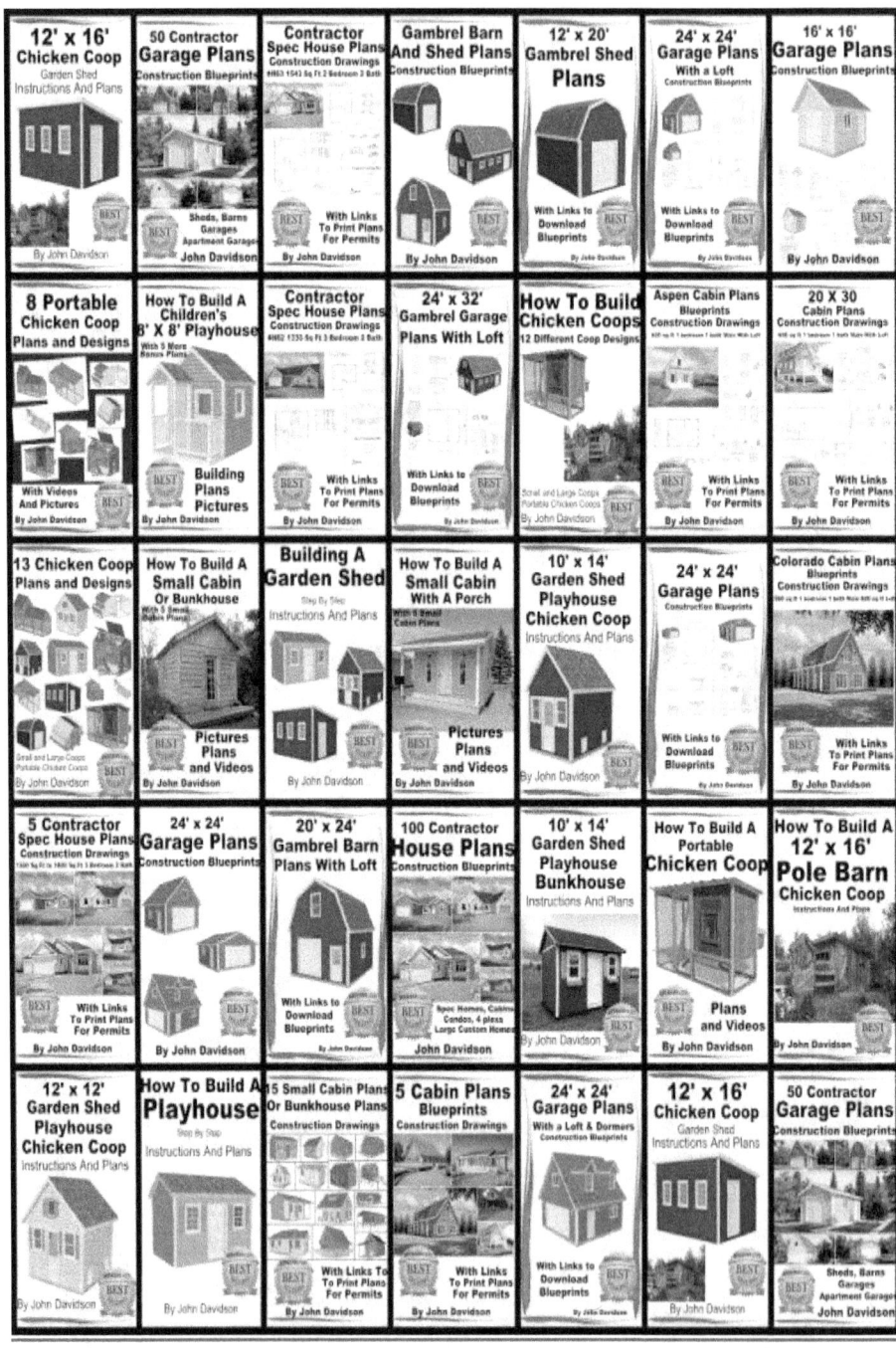

Entrepreneur Book Series

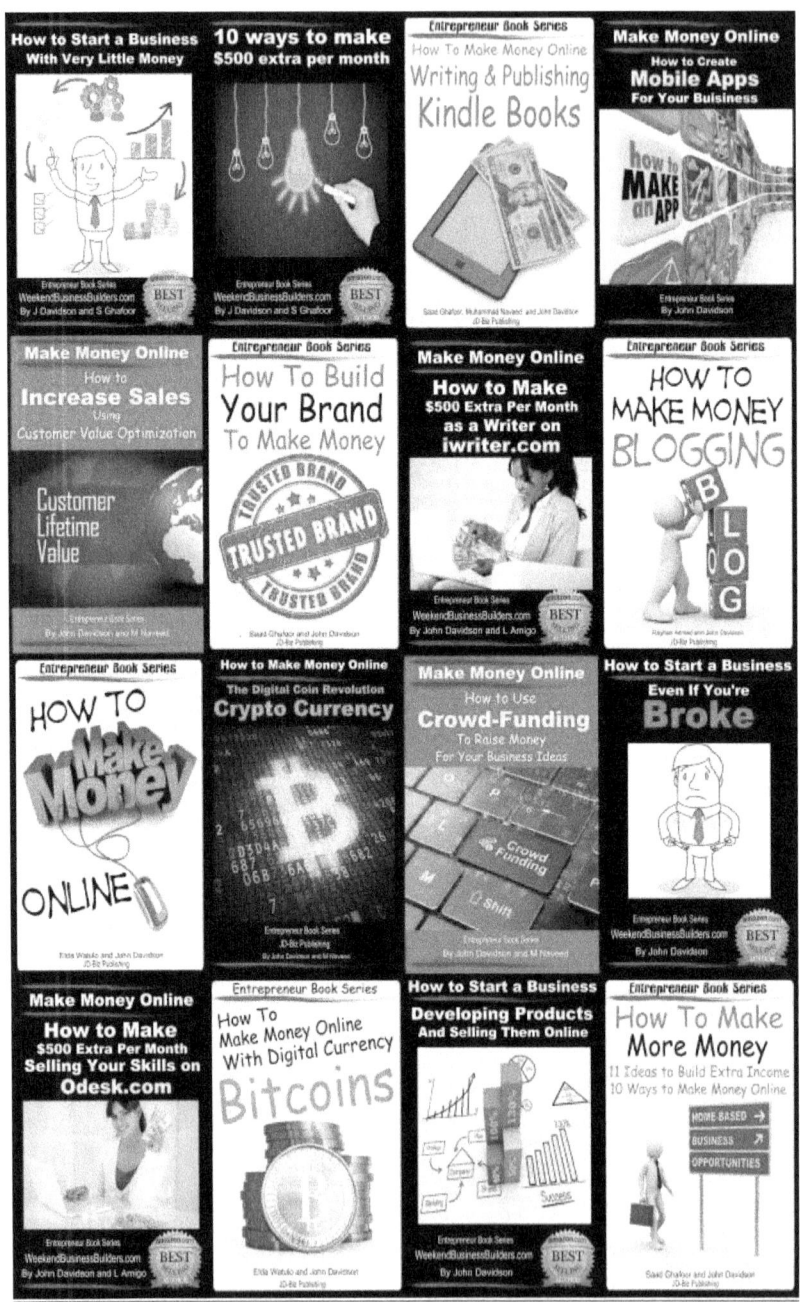

Our books are available at

1. Amazon.com

2. Barnes and Noble

3. Itunes

4. Kobo

5. Smashwords

6. Google Play Books

Publisher

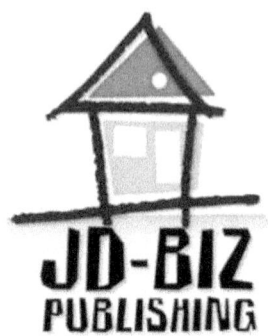

JD-Biz Corp

P O Box 374

Mendon, Utah 84325

http://www.jd-biz.com/

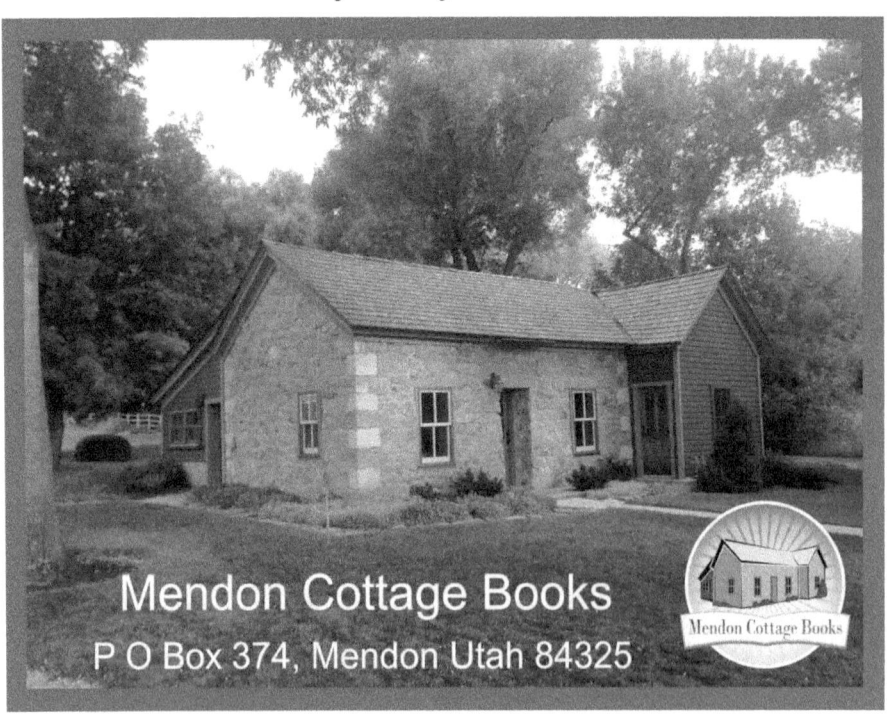

Mendon Cottage Books

P O Box 374, Mendon Utah 84325

www.ingramcontent.com/pod-product-compliance
Lightning Source LLC
Chambersburg PA
CBHW061802280526
45787CB00003BA/1452